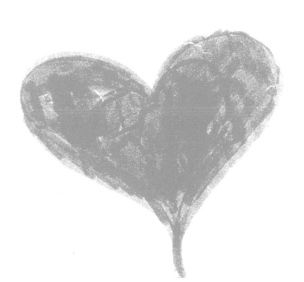

The Dougy Center for Grieving Children

3909 S.E. 52nd Avenue

P.O. Box 86852 Portland, OR 97286

Phone: 503-775-5683

Fax: 503-777-3097

Email: help@dougy.org

Website: www.dougy.org

Written and printed in the United States of America.

ISBN: 1-890534-01-3

Revised 9/2006

Our Mission

The mission of The Dougy Center for Grieving Children is to provide to families in Portland and the surrounding region loving support in a safe place where children, teens and their families grieving a death can share their experiences as they move through their healing process. Through our National Center for Grieving Children & Families we also provide support and training locally, nationally and internationally to individuals and organizations seeking to assist children in grief.

The Dougy Center is supported solely through private support from individuals, foundations and companies, and receives no state or federal funding. The Dougy Center does not charge a fee for its services.

Table of Contents

Development of this guidebook was
made possible through a grant from the
Meyer Memorial Trust

Introduction

This guidebook has been developed by The Dougy Center, The National Center for Grieving Children & Families. Since 1983, the Center has worked with thousands of children, teens and their adult family members who have experienced the death of a parent, adult caregiver, sibling or teen friend. It is written for you—teachers and school personnel who come in direct, daily contact with grieving students.

Children and teens currently spend an average of six hours a day, 30 hours a week, in school. One out of every 750 youth of high-school age die each year and one child in 20 will have a parent die before he or she graduates from high school. According to U.S. Census Bureau statistics released in December 1995, 830,000 children and teens in the United States live with a widowed parent. That represents about 1% of the childhood population, and indicates that in every school a number of students are, or will be, grieving a death.

As a teacher, you have the opportunity to touch children's lives in a very special way. Your actions can have a lifelong impact. When a death influences the lives of your students, you, and your school, can provide an environment which encourages healing and support.

In the school community, everyone is impacted in one way or another by the grieving process. In your classroom, you can use subjects such as the death of a classroom pet or even the changing of the seasons as an opportunity to discuss and amplify issues around death. You have the ability to educate your students about healthy grief and ways to be supportive and empathic to a grieving person. By seizing these teachable moments, the school community will be a better place for all who are affected by the experience.

At The Dougy Center we are often called upon to help a school community cope after a death. During these interventions we teach the faculty what they may expect from grieving students and staff, as well as effective ways to support them. Sometimes we meet with the students or parents who are directly impacted by a death. Those schools that address the death directly, talk about concerns and allow for grieving and plan memorials are better able to facilitate students' healing through a healthy grief process.

Too often our society fails to support young people and adults after a death. Those grieving may experience isolation and misunderstanding because people pressure them to move on, put the experience behind them and get on with life. Without processing feelings and thoughts of loss and grief, individuals cannot integrate the loss into their lives.

Keeping feelings inside and pushing away disturbing thoughts does not facilitate healing. The result may be social, physical, emotional, cognitive and spiritual problems for those grieving—now and in the future.

The information presented in this guide has been compiled from the experiences of the children, their parents and school staff with whom we have worked since 1983.

This book is dedicated to the thousands of children, teens, and adults who have courageously shared their pain, their stories and their healing. They, the grievers, have been our best teachers at The Dougy Center.

What is Grief?

Many people believe that grief is the outward display of feelings about a significant loss—that grief is something you can observe. If a child isn't visibly tearful, sad or crying, people may assume that he/she is not grieving. This common, yet incorrect belief, leads to many problems when it comes to understanding and helping a grieving person. It is especially true for a child or teen, whose grief experience is very different from that of an adult.

Grief is the internal anguish bereaved persons feel in reaction to a loss that they have experienced. For purposes of this guidebook, the specific loss we are referring to is a death. Internal responses to death may include:

- Emotions such as anger, guilt, relief, fear and sadness
- Thought processes like understanding and believing that the person is gone
- Physical responses such as sleeplessness, stomachaches, headaches or loss of appetite
- Spiritual questioning about the meaning of life and the existence and nature of God

Grieving may or may not "show" on the outside. Keep in mind that a child who is not crying can still be quite sad. And a teen who does not visibly appear depressed might actually be hurting deeply.

Children and teens are still developing their capacities for understanding and coping with life and death. When someone close to them dies, it is a new experience and they are typically ill-prepared for its impact. Adults may also be unprepared to deal with their own responses to death. Therefore, it is often hard for them to cope with what the children and teens close to them are going through.

"Children and teens may express their grieving outwardly, and they may not."

When students experience death, they may express their grieving outwardly, and they may not. Their actions may be direct and intentional: talking about how they feel, writing poetry or simply crying. Or they may be indirect: withdrawing, risk-taking behaviors, attempting to be "perfect."

The external behaviors that a grieving child or teen exhibits are termed "mourning." All children and teens who have been

3

impacted by a death are grieving; they may or may not mourn. In an attempt to help grieving students, this distinction is a critical one. We should not assume that individuals are not grieving because we cannot "see" a reaction.

Six Basic Concepts of Grief

1 Grief is a natural reaction to loss.

Grief is a natural reaction to loss. When a person dies, individuals impacted by the death experience emotional and physical reactions. This is true for infants through adults, although the reactions will vary from person to person. Grief does not feel natural, in part, because we cannot necessarily control our emotions or other responses. The sense of being out of control may be overwhelming or frightening. However, grieving is natural, normal and healthy for bereaved students and adults.

2 Each student's grief experience is unique.

While many theories and models of the grieving process provide a helpful framework of tasks or stages of grieving, the path itself is a lonely, solitary and unique one for every individual. No book, article or grief therapist can predict or prescribe exactly what a student or an adult will—or should—encounter on this path. Those who wish to assist people in grief do so best by walking with them along the path, in the role of listener and learner, allowing the griever to teach about his or her unique grief journey.

"It is important to remember that each student will express grief in a personal way."

3 There are no "right" and "wrong" ways to grieve.

Coping with the death of someone does not follow a set pattern or set of rules. There is no "right" or "wrong" way to grieve. There are, however, "helpful" choices and behaviors that are constructive and life-affirming. Other responses are "unhelpful," destructive or even harmful, causing long-term complications. The sheer pain of loss often feels "crazy." It may be challenging to decide which thoughts, feelings and actions are helpful, and which are not.

Following a death, grieving students get plenty of advice from others about what they should and shouldn't do, feel, think and believe. What is often more helpful than advice is non-judgmental listening. This can help grieving students sort through the options and alternatives.

4 Every death is different and will be experienced by your students in differing ways.

Students react differently to the death of a parent, sibling, friend, teacher or principal. It makes sense—each relationship meets different needs and is uniquely personal. Some of the grief literature talks about loss in an almost competitive way as if some losses are worse than others. You may read that the death of a child is "the worst loss." Or that suicide is the hardest to "get over." Comparisons about which death is the worst are not helpful and may lead to unrealistic expectations or demands. While a student may speak for herself about how she experienced different losses, one cannot categorically say that any loss is worse than or easier than another. Each person's way should be honored as his or her way of coping with the death.

"I've had teachers say you've got to go on, you've got to get over this. I just want to shout 'You're wrong! Grief never ends.' I don't care what they say."

—Philip, 13

5 The grieving process is influenced by a multitude of factors.

There are many factors that influence a student's reaction to a death. They include the following:

- Social support systems available to the student (family, school, community, friends)
- The nature of the death and how the student interprets it
- Status of "unfinished business" between the student and the person who died
- The previous nature of the relationship
- The emotional and developmental age of the student
- Community views on the death (Stigmatized deaths such as homicides, suicides and AIDS are often looked at very differently from deaths by illness or accident)

6 Grieving never ends. It is something the student will never "get over."

This is perhaps one of the least understood aspects of grief in our society. It seems that most people are anxious for us to put the loss behind us, to go on, to get over it. When a person dies, the death leaves a vacuum in the lives of those left behind. Life is never the same again. This doesn't mean that life can never again be joyful, or that the experience of loss cannot be transformed into something positive. But grief does not have a magical ending time. People comment on the pangs of grief 40, 50 or 60 years after a death. For the student, the grieving process will be re-experienced in some new way at each developmental level or experience of personal accomplishment.

How Bereaved Students Grieve

Grieving is very hard work for students. It influences all areas of the student's life—academic, social, physical, emotional, spiritual and behavioral. Students cannot control where or when they will be affected by their grief. Although some students will be able to talk about their feelings, many others may express their grief through their behavior and play. You may see a student who becomes more aggressive on the playground or who shows no fear; another who becomes withdrawn and quiet. Still others may show grief with physical symptoms such as stomachaches or headaches. Because each student grieves differently, we cannot predict how an individual student will grieve.

It is important to remember that many grieving students will focus on their grief first and school work second. They could not change this response, even if they wanted to. Teachers who allow their students time and support for healing provide a real gift to them. Those who tell students to "just get over it" or say "you have been grieving long enough" can create additional problems. It is important to remember that each student will express grief in a personal way. Some students will exhibit several of the behaviors listed and others may show none.

Common Responses of the Grieving Child or Teen

Academic

- Inability to focus or concentrate
- Failing or declining grades
- Incomplete work, or poor quality of work
- Increased absences or reluctance to go to school
- Forgetfulness, memory loss
- Over achievement, trying to be perfect
- Language errors and word-finding problems
- Inattentiveness
- Daydreaming

"Teachers who allow their students time and support for healing provide a real gift to them."

Behavioral

- Noisy outbursts, disruptive behaviors
- Aggressive behaviors, frequent fighting
- Non-compliance to requests
- Increase in risk-taking or unsafe behaviors
- "Hyperactive-like" behavior
- Isolation or withdrawal
- Regressive behaviors to a time when things felt more safe and in control
- High need for attention
- A need for checking in on surviving parent(s)

Emotional

- Insecurity, issues of abandonment, safety concerns
- Concern about being treated differently from others
- Fear, guilt, anger, rage, regret, sadness, confusion
- "I don't care" attitude
- Depression, hopelessness, intense sadness
- Overly sensitive, frequently tearful, irritable
- Appears unaffected by the death
- Preoccupation with death, wanting details
- Recurring thoughts of death or suicide

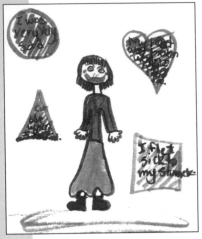

Social
- Withdrawal from friends
- Withdrawal from activities or sports
- Use of drugs or alcohol
- Changes in relationships with teachers and peers
- Changes in family roles (e.g. taking on the role of a deceased parent)
- Wanting to be physically close to safe adults
- Sexual acting out
- Stealing, shoplifting
- Difficulty with being in a group or crowd

Physical
- Stomachaches, headaches, heartaches
- Frequent accidents or injuries
- Increased requests to visit the nurse
- Nightmares, dreams or sleep difficulties
- Loss of appetite or increased eating
- Low energy, weakness
- Hives, rashes, itching
- Nausea, or upset stomach
- Increased illnesses, low resistance to colds, flu
- Rapid heart beat

Spiritual
- Anger at God
- Questions of "Why me?" and "Why now?"
- Questions about the meaning of life
- Confusion about where the person is who died
- Feelings of being alone in the universe
- Doubting or questioning previous beliefs
- Sense of meaninglessness about the future
- Change in values, questioning what is important

How to Tell When Students Need Additional Help

Most children and teens are "in and out" of their grief. They experience sadness, anger and fear, but also are able to have fun and engage in activities. This is a normal grief response. Prolonged or chronic depression, anger, withdrawal or fear over a period of several months may indicate that the student needs professional help in dealing with the loss.

If a child or teen displays severe reactions or you notice disturbing changes in behavior, professional intervention should be sought. Although it is not unusual for children or teens to talk about wanting to join the deceased, or to die, any signs of suicidal talk or other self-destructive behavior or language should be taken seriously. The student should be referred for an evaluation. If a child or teen is experiencing physical pain or problems and doctors have not found an organic reason for the pain, professional counseling or therapy may be helpful. Having physical symptoms following a death is not unusual. However, if they become problematic or debilitating, or persist over time, professional help by a qualified mental health professional should be sought.

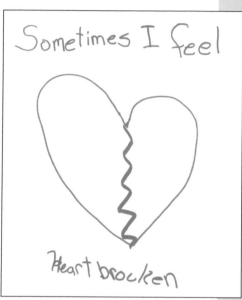

"Prolonged or chronic depression, anger, withdrawal or fear over a period of several months may indicate that the student needs professional help in dealing with the loss."

Behaviors that suggest complications in the grieving process and indicate the need for a referral to a mental health professional include:

- Suicidal thoughts or behaviors
- Chronic physical symptoms without organic findings
- Depression with impaired self-esteem

- Persistent denial of the death with delayed or absent grieving
- Progressive isolation and lack of interest in any activity
- Resistant anger and hostility
- Intense preoccupation with memories of the deceased
- Taking on the symptoms of the deceased
- Prolonged changes in typical behavior
- The use of alcohol and/or other drugs
- Prolonged feelings of guilt or responsibility for the death
- Major and continued changes in sleeping or eating patterns
- Risk-taking behaviors that may include identifying with the deceased in unsafe ways

Developmental Issues of Grieving Students

The developmental level of the students, rather than chronological age, will determine the ways that they will proceed in their grief journey. The following guidelines are for the teacher or counselor. If the student does not match his or her appropriate age or developmental level, it does not mean that the student has a problem or is doing something wrong. It is important to remember that each student grieves in his or her own way and on his or her own timeline.

The Grieving Infant and Toddler

Infants and toddlers who are grieving have an intuitive sense that something very serious has happened, even if they don't fully understand what it is. They are able to read the expressions and sense the emotions in their environment. Their reactions are sensory and physical. Any child old enough to smile or express emotional reaction is old enough to grieve. Infants and toddlers don't have sophisticated verbal skills, but they will still express their grief through their behaviors and play.

Common Behaviors to Expect
- General anxiety
- Crying
- Sleeplessness
- Excessive sleeping

- Stomach problems
- Clinginess, needing to be held
- Separation anxiety
- Biting
- Throwing things
- Regression through baby talk, bed-wetting
- Irritability
- Temper tantrums
- Clumsiness

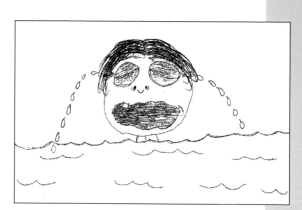

How to Help

- Lots of holding, additional nurturing and physical contact
- A consistent routine, including regular meal and bed times
- Rules and limits that are concrete and specific
- Short, truthful statements about what has happened
- Making time for play, both physical and imaginative

The Grieving Preschool Child

Preschool children are naturally egocentric. They believe that the world revolves around them and that they cause things to happen. Without a developed cognitive understanding of death, they often experience death as abandonment. Their "magical thinking" may lead them to believe that they have somehow caused the death, or can bring the deceased back. Their grief responses are usually intense but brief, and often experienced at specific times such as missing daddy at bedtime when he tucked them in bed. Because pre-school children learn by repetition, they will ask repeatedly about the death. They also learn by play, and their main grief work will be accomplished through playing rather than talking.

Frequently, grieving preschoolers will regress to earlier behaviors.

Common Behaviors to Expect

- Changes in eating and sleeping patterns
- Wanting to be dressed or fed
- Thumb sucking

- Baby talk
- Wanting a bottle
- Bed wetting
- General irritability
- Concerns about safety and abandonment
- General confusion

How To Help
- Use simple, honest answers
- Be prepared to answer the same questions over and over
- Include the child in the rituals around the death
- Support the child in his or her play
- Allow for anger and physical expression
- Maintain consistent structure and routines
- Allow the child to act younger for a while
- Hold and nurture the child, giving lots of physical attention
- Encourage and allow for fun and happy times
- Have books and posters on death and grief available
- Have toys, dress-ups and other props which facilitate expression during play time
- Address grief issues in a group setting without focusing on the grieving child, like reading a story or using a persona doll
- Model by sharing personal anecdotes as appropriate

"Be prepared to answer the same questions over and over."

The Grieving Elementary School Student

Elementary-aged students are concrete thinkers who are beginning to develop logical thinking patterns along with increased language and cognitive ability. After a death, they begin questioning how their lives will be different, what will be the same, and how one knows the person is really dead. They are usually interested in how the body works and ask specific questions like: "Did his blood get all over the windshield?" or "Will her hair fall out now that she's dead?" It is not unusual for their questions and play to be graphic and gory, displaying a fear of bodily harm and mutilation. Although their discussions and play can be unsettling to teachers and parents, it is important to give simple, honest answers to their questions.

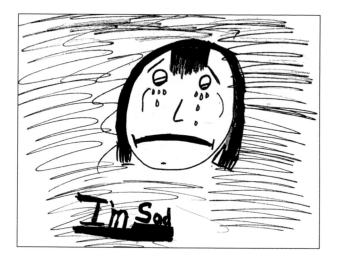

The overwhelming concern with the body and what is happening to it may bring about the desire to be with the deceased person. For example, it is not unusual for children to say things like, "I wish I was dead so I could be with daddy." Statements like this do not necessarily mean the child is suicidal or really wants to die; rather, they are most often expressions of deep longing for the deceased. However, any time a child talks about wanting to die, it should be taken seriously and explored. Discerning whether the child is expressing a normal, common desire to be with the lost loved one, or is truly at risk of endangering their own life may be difficult. If you have any concerns, request professional intervention immediately.

While 6 to 12 year olds want to see death as reversible, they are also beginning to understand that it is final. Because they are beginning to understand the permanence of the death, they may begin to worry about their own and others' deaths. They often perceive death as a punishment for something they did, and therefore, they associate guilt with death.

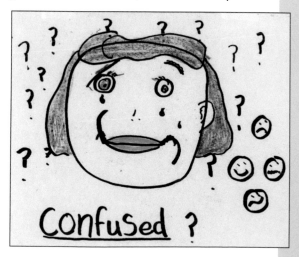

They may think, "If only I'd been a better daughter or son, maybe my mom would still be alive." They are beginning to become more socially aware, and look to others to see if they are acting or responding correctly. The family is still the main security and support, but their role in the family has changed and they need to figure out what their new role is.

Because school is such an integral part of the student's life, and because the academic expectations are increasing, you may notice that grieving students have difficulty attending, staying focused, remembering what was said and completing assignments. These are normal grief responses and should be expected and planned for. Students may also appear withdrawn or depressed. Many grieving students have difficulty getting to sleep, wake up during the night, have night terrors or awaken very early. Teachers may notice these students come to school tired.

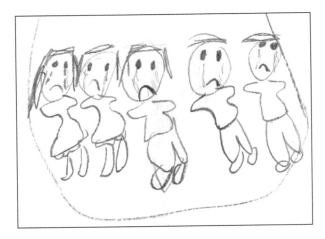

Common Behaviors to Expect
- Regression to earlier behaviors
- Fighting, anger
- Difficulty in paying attention and concentrating
- Daydreaming
- Not completing homework or assignments
- Sleepiness
- Withdrawal

How to Help

- Answer questions as clearly and accurately as possible
- Provide art, journal, music and movement activities
- Make time for physical outlets: sports, games, walks, etc.
- Help the student identify and use support systems
- Work with the student around academic assignments
- Encourage the student to take a break and have some alone time
- Allow for expression of feelings and emotions
- Maintain routines and structure but allow for flexibility
- Give the student choices whenever possible
- Let the student know you care and are thinking about her
- Assign the student a buddy who can work with her
- Create a "safe space" where a student can go when needed

The Grieving Middle School Student

Middle school students are, under the best conditions, experiencing a great deal of turmoil due to the physical and hormonal changes in their bodies. Grieving students must deal with the additional stress of the grief process. Because of the many physical changes, pre-adolescents tend to have a variety of physical symptoms such as headaches, stomach problems, sleep disturbances and changes in eating patterns.

They generally experience a range of emotional reactions. In addition, they may be beginning to get their primary support from friends rather than family, as in the past. The normal process of moving away from family toward friends for support is altered when a death impacts them. They want very much to be like their peers and not to be treated differently just because of the death in their family. They often become confused about how and from whom they can get their support.

Although preteen students are much more verbal and process information at a higher level, physical outlets are still very important to the preteen student. They comprehend that death is final and unavoidable. This may provoke feelings of helplessness and hopelessness, and may increase risk-taking behaviors. These students are apt to exhibit concerns about the survivors and what their future holds.

Common Behaviors to Expect

- Argumentative
- Withdrawal, sullenness
- Anger, fighting
- Sleepiness
- Lack of concentration and attentiveness
- Risk-taking behaviors (drugs, sexual acting out, stealing)
- Unpredictable ups and downs, or moodiness
- Erratic, inconsistent reactions

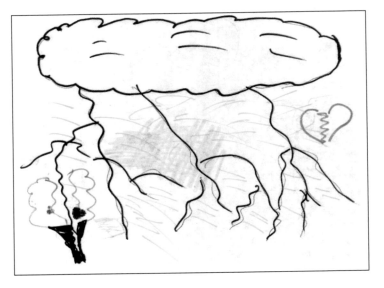

How to Help

- Expect and accept mood swings
- Provide a supportive environment where the student can share, when needed
- Anticipate increased physical concerns, including illness and body aches and pains
- Allow the student choices, including with whom and how she gets support
- Encourage participation in a support group
- Allow flexibility in completing school work

The Grieving High School Student

High school students are often philosophical about life and death and believe that death won't happen to them. While functioning at the formal operational stage of cognitive development, they appear to use "adult" approaches of problem solving and abstract thinking in dealing with their grief. However, it is important to remember that high school students are not yet adults. In their attempts to make sense of the world and what has happened to them, you may see depression, denial, anger, risk-taking and acting-out behaviors. You may see teens fighting against their vulnerability because they want very much to be independent. It is not unusual for people to assume that a teen will become responsible for the family. A boy whose father 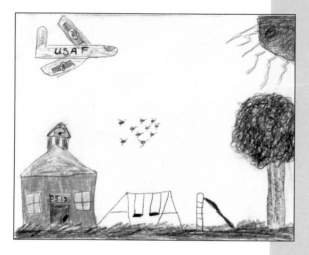 has died may be told that he is now "the man of the family." Or, a girl whose mother has died may find out that she is expected to "take care" of her dad and brothers.

After her brother died, a 15 year old dropped out of school for three months and never left the house. She spent a lot of time wearing his clothes and sitting in his closet. The parents were terrified, but a wise therapist said "be patient with her, she is grieving her way." When she returned to school she resumed her role as a good student.

Common Behaviors to Expect

- Withdrawal from parents and other adults
- Angry outbursts
- Increased risk-taking behaviors (substances, reckless driving, sexual behaviors)

17

- Pushing the limits of rules
- Lack of concentration; inability to focus
- Hanging out with a small group of friends
- Sad face, evidence of crying
- Sleepiness, exhaustion

How to Help

- Allow for regression and dependency
- Encourage expression of feelings such as sorrow, anger, guilt, regret
- Understand and allow for variation in maturity level
- Answer questions honestly and provide factual information
- Model appropriate responses, showing the students your own grief
- Avoid power struggles and allow choices
- Help students understand and resolve feelings of helplessness
- Assist students with plans for completion of assignments
- Allow for some flexibility in assignments, e.g. be willing to adapt assignments to topics relevant to the student's current experience

How Teachers Can Help Grieving Students

Your Important Role In Helping Students Cope with a Death

Perhaps you feel ill-prepared and somewhat overwhelmed at the prospect of helping your students cope with a death. If so, you're not alone. You already have plenty of responsibilities without adding the unique challenges of assisting a grieving student. Most likely in your education as a teacher, you did not receive any training in helping your students cope with death.

If this is true for you, please understand that the most important qualities for assisting a grieving student are ones that you already have: good listening skills and the ability to understand what your students are dealing with.

You have the ability to significantly alter a student's life forever in the ways you choose to respond when he or she is deeply affected by a death. Virtually all of the students we have worked with over the years have talked about teachers who were present and helpful to them, as well as those who were not. If you are able to travel with the student on her journey, you will personally gain a great deal and will provide a special gift to a griever.

Groundwork for Dealing with Grieving Students in Your Class

The following steps help ensure that a grieving student is comfortable with your approach to providing support. They also help you prepare your class for making the grieving student feel comfortable and supported:

First, ask the student what she wants the class to know about the death, funeral arrangements, etc.

If possible, call the family prior to her return to school so that you can provide support and let her know you are thinking of her and want to help make her return to school as helpful as possible.

Talk to your class about how grief affects people and encourage them to share how they feel.

One way to do this is to discuss what other types of losses or deaths the students in your class have experienced, and what helped them cope. It is important to provide a safe environment where students in your class can talk about how they're feeling and have the opportunity to ask questions. You can encourage constructive outlets for the expression of feelings through art, journal writing or other activities.

Discuss how difficult it may be for their classmate to return to school, and how they may be of help.

You can ask your class for ideas about how they would like others to treat them if they were returning to school after a death, pointing out differences in preference. Some students would like to be left alone; others want the circumstances discussed freely.

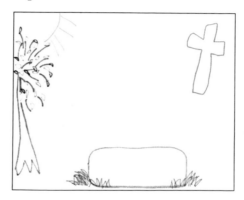

Most grieving students say that they want everyone to treat them the same way that they were treated before. As a rule, they don't like people being "extra nice." While students usually say they don't want to be in the spotlight, they also don't want people acting like nothing happened.

Provide a way for your class to reach out to the grieving classmate and his or her family.

One of the ways that students can reach out is by sending cards or pictures to the child and family, letting them know the class is thinking of them. If students in your class knew the person who died, they could share memories of that person. Many students learn new things about their family member who died through memories shared by friends and acquaintances. These shared memories are important because they provide a meaningful remembrance of a loved one.

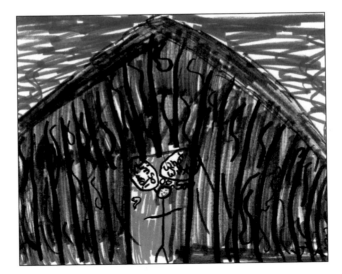

Provide flexibility and support to your grieving student upon his or her return to class.

Recognize that your student will have difficulty concentrating and focusing on school work. Allow the bereaved student to leave the class when she is needing some quiet or alone time. Make sure that the student has a person available to talk with, such as the school counselor.

Ongoing Support for Grieving Students and Classmates

Be a Good Listener

What grieving students find most helpful is a safe, trusted person, who will listen to them. They want to tell their story, share their fears and concerns and just be with a safe adult when they need to be quiet. Grieving students have taught us that they don't want to be treated differently, yet they are different. Ask your students to explain to you what happened and reflect back to them what they said. Have them tell you what they need and what would be helpful to them, giving them choices and suggestions. They usually will be able to tell you what they want.

"The most important qualities for assisting a grieving student are ones that you already have: good listening skills and the ability to understand where your students are coming from."

Follow Routines

During the grief process it is helpful for bereaved students to know that there is a structure and routine to their day. When they know what to expect, they can let go of worrying about what will happen next. This allows them the emotional energy that they need to work on their grief. Routines provide a sense of safety, which is very comforting to the grieving student. It is important to remember that there will be times when it is best to give up the planned activity and use a teachable moment to allow students to talk about the death or to remember the person who died. These moments cannot always be planned, but can be very valuable learning experiences for the class. Be careful not to become rigid with regard to routines.

"It was terrible that our teacher made us take our final exam the day after our friend was killed. We couldn't even think, let alone concentrate on a test."

—*Sally, 14*

Set Limits

Along with routines, it is important to set limits for students. Limits help provide a safe and consistent environment. Just because students are grieving does not mean that the rules do not apply.

When grieving, students may experience lapses in concentration or exhibit risk-taking behavior. Setting clear limits provides a more secure and safe environment for everyone under these circumstances. Often people allow the grieving child to do anything he or she wants, which generally is not helpful. What she may want and need most is to have someone tell her what to do.

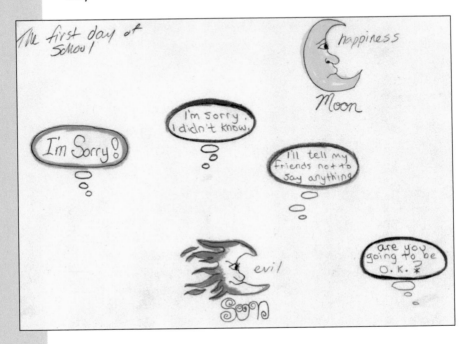

Be Aware Of and Sensitive to "Trigger" Events

As the grieving student returns to class, there will be times when something will trigger thoughts or feelings about the deceased person. These triggers may include any or all of the five senses: seeing a person who looks like the deceased, hearing a song or other sound, smelling a favorite cologne, tasting something the person loved or just remembering something about that person.

When the student remembers something about the deceased, it often elicits some type of response. Individuals have no control over when they will be triggered, or how strong their reaction will be. These moments are often embarrassing for the student. When this occurs it is helpful to allow the student some private time and to have a compassionate listener available if the student needs one. Allow the student to express her feelings without trying to talk her out of them or "fix things." Remember that any feeling is okay; they are not right or wrong, good or bad.

After a sudden fatal heart attack of a fifth-grade teacher, the students all remembered the cologne that the teacher always wore. When one of his students smelled the scent while at a restaurant, she looked around for her teacher. These "trigger" events may happen in your classroom, or at any time.

Certain school activities and holidays can create strong reactions for a grieving student.

Holidays are often difficult because they bring up memories, sadness that the person is not there, or the fact that the student is different from her friends. Father's Day, Mother's Day and activities such as Father/Daughter dances, Mother/Daughter teas and even Parent Night can put the student in a difficult position. The children at The Dougy Center ask questions such as, "How can you make a Mother's Day card when your mom is dead?" or "I don't have a father to take me to the dance." On such occasions the student feels left out, embarrassed, angry or not sure what to do. If you are sensitive to these potential issues, you can suggest alternatives for the student. For example, you could suggest making a Father's Day memory card for a deceased father, including the special things that they did together.

After a death, many students feel confused or awkward about special days and how to handle them. They question if they should still celebrate the birthday of the deceased. Birthdays, holidays and anniversaries are especially hard for grieving students because they do not want to be different or stand out, yet they are faced with just that reality. Using the name of the deceased and sharing memories about the person is helpful to the grieving student. On the anniversary date of the death, children often have strong reactions. It is important to acknowledge the date and let the student know that you are thinking of them during this difficult time.

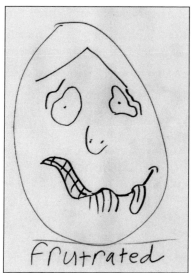

23

Steps You Can Take to Help

- Tell the truth, use accurate words such as died, killed, suicided
- Listen without judgment
- Say something that acknowledges you care and know about the death, like "I'm sorry about your mom's death, and I would like to help in any way I can." (Some kids say they don't like people to say they're sorry because it's not their fault)
- Talk about the person who died, using their name and sharing memories
- Provide structure and routine with flexibility as needed
- Seize those special moments that may arise in class to teach about grief
- Know that you can't take away the pain, fear, aloneness or feeling of being different. And understand that your role is not to get rid of those feelings, but to provide a safe atmosphere where they can be expressed

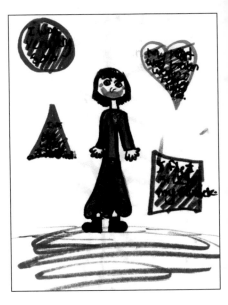

- Provide a structured, safe environment for grief
- Comprehend that the student's life has changed forever, and that it will never be the same
- Allow for grief, sorrow, anger, other feelings
- Provide a support group in the school for grieving students
- With young children, give concrete examples about death. For example, you can say that when a person dies they don't have to go to the bathroom; they don't get cold or hungry; they don't sleep or think; they don't get scared, etc. Help students understand that a dead body does not do what a live body does

Common Mistakes: Words and Actions to Avoid

The following words and actions can be harmful to children and teens.

- DO NOT suggest that the student has grieved long enough
- DO NOT indicate that the student should get over it and move on
- DO NOT expect the student to complete all assignments on a timely basis
- DO NOT act as if nothing has happened
- DO NOT say things like:
  "It could be worse, you still have one brother"
  "I know how you feel"
  "You'll be stronger because of this"

Taking Care of Yourself

As a teacher, there may be many occasions when you experience exhaustion and sadness in working with your students over difficult situations that they are facing. Watching students cope with a death is a difficult, painful and draining journey. Many teachers we have worked with have expressed frustration about having to deal with such difficult situations without adequate training to prepare them. We suggest that you urge your school administrators to include sessions on dealing with death in the classroom as part of your ongoing training programs.

You should also be aware that when a death occurs, it can bring up personal feelings about losses and deaths from your own past. Many teachers are uncomfortable talking about death and therefore choose not to talk with others about their feelings. Until you've worked on your own unresolved issues about death, it will be difficult for you to effectively work with your students.

Ways to Take Care of Yourself After a Death Include:

- Making time to talk with other staff members about grieving students
- Talking with those you trust about your own feelings
- Remembering that grief issues take time to process and that there is no set time frame
- Seeking professional support when necessary
- Getting physical activity, sleep and reflective time
- Drinking plenty of water

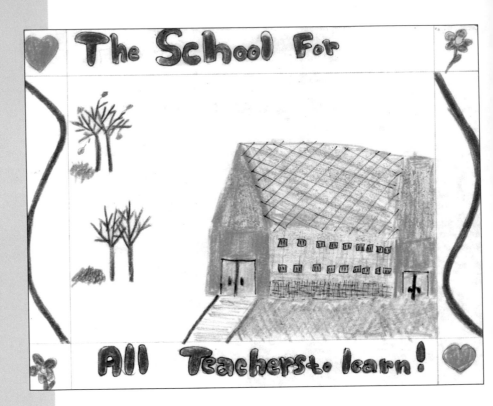

Responding to a School-Related Death

What Administrators and Teachers Should Do

It is important for the school community to acknowledge the death of one of their students or staff members, as well as the death of a student's family member. This emphasizes the importance of every person's life and models respect for life. It gives students a chance to say goodbye and it begins the healing journey.

When a student or teacher in your school dies, everyone in your school community is affected. It is important to tell the staff and students as soon as possible, in a personal way. In elementary schools or smaller schools, the principal or school counselor can go to each classroom and, along with the classroom teacher, tell the students the news. **Do not announce the news over the PA system or in a large assembly.** Each student will respond differently and it is usually very difficult to predict who will react strongly and who will not react at all. In the security of the classroom each student can feel safe to react, ask questions, talk about the impact of the news and express emotions and thoughts.

Many schools have set up phone trees to inform school personnel in emergencies prior to the start of the school day, or on weekends. If possible, all school personnel should be contacted about a death prior to the start of the school day. The Dougy Center's guidebook for school administrators, *When Death Impacts Your School: A Guide for School Administrators*, provides step-by-step suggestions for what the school administration should do following a death.

Some staff members may believe that if the school personnel don't say anything about the death, it won't be an issue for the students. Others think that only those students who are "directly involved" with the person, such as students in his or her classes, should be told. We have found that it is important to inform all students, parents and staff about a death. All of the students will hear about the death, at recess, on the playground, in the bathroom or the halls. Hearing correct information from a caring adult who can provide support is important for students. It is a much better proactive response than just reacting.

When sharing the news with the students, we suggest that you have a written statement with the facts so that all students get the same information. The information should be factual, honest and use correct words such as dead, killed, died by suicide or murdered. Words that are not helpful to students include phrases such as: "She passed on." "We lost him." "She expired." "She went to her final resting place." Or "God took him." Say "Sam died last night," not "We lost Sam last night."

All deaths should be treated in a consistent manner, whether it is the death of a football star or gang member; from cancer or by suicide. That is, if a letter informing parents of the death of a student due to a car accident is sent home, one should also be sent home following the suicide of a student. If an assembly is held to memorialize a football player stricken with cancer, one should also be held to memorialize a gang member killed in a drive-by shooting.

Occasionally, school personnel have encountered difficulties with students making "shrines" out of lockers. Or students may inadvertently block hallways because they are convening at a deceased classmate's locker. Bear in mind that these young people are hurting. As adults, we should be sensitive to their needs while also maintaining order. Rather than simply taking down pictures, notes or drawings placed on a student's locker and demanding that students disperse, provide a time to meet with the students affected and develop a compromise. For example, the school could allow a display case to be used to exhibit notes, cards and expressions collected at the student's locker for a specific time.

If a student or teacher has died, there should be a period of time when his or her desk or locker remains unchanged. The visual reminder often helps students with their grieving. Whisking a student's desk out of the class immediately minimizes the impact of the student's life on others. In general, it is a good idea to involve the students in the class around these decisions, asking them what they'd like to see done with the desk, locker, etc.

It is important to call or send a letter to parents of your students to inform them of the news of a death, what was shared with the students and common grief responses to expect. School administrators may wish to schedule an evening meeting for parents. This provides a forum for parents to discuss their concerns, ask questions and participate in an open discussion about the death and its effect on their children.

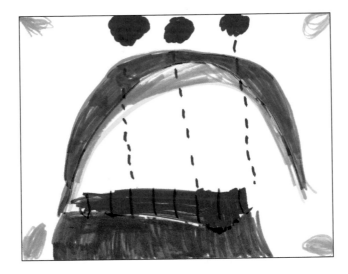

How to Tell Students About a Death

- Have students sit in a circle on the floor or in chairs rather than at their desks. This tends to provide an environment in which students may be better able to share their feelings and questions.

- Ask students if they know what happened. Ask them how they found out. At this point allow them to share what they know or think without correcting them.

- Share the information that you have about the death directly and honestly.

- Allow students to ask questions. Answer questions as best you can, knowing it is okay to say "I don't know" when you don't have the answers.
- Allow students to share their experiences and feelings about the death as well as about other deaths that they have experienced.
- Have students share memories of the deceased person.
- Talk about a memorial and ways to remember the person.
- Discuss common grief responses that a student might experience, such as difficulty concentrating, sudden emotional reactions or strong feelings of anger or sadness.
- Talk about okay ways to handle the grief reactions.
- Have an art activity or something physical to do after the sharing.
- Provide a safe room where students can go if they need some alone time, want to talk to someone or just want to be away from the class for a period of time.

Remember that grief is a process, not an event—and that healing takes time. Students are not always able to control their emotions and reactions. These feelings often come up very suddenly and unexpectedly at inconvenient times. Be flexible.

School-Sponsored Activities in Response to a Death

Your school should have a policy about school memorials. If the school decides to have a memorial, allow students to participate in the planning whenever possible, especially those students who knew the deceased. This may include students from the class of the deceased, a sports team or a group of friends. The process of planning allows the students to feel ownership of the process and is often a healing experience for the students. All students in the school should be invited, allowing them to make a choice about attendance.

There are many ways in which to remember a person from the school community. If you hold a schoolwide memorial, it could include:

- Selected students sharing memories
- A display of pictures, drawings, cards and notes
- The sharing of a favorite song
- A candle-lighting ceremony
- A book for the family of letters, pictures and memories

In addition to or in place of a memorial service, other ways to commemorate the person could include:

- Placing a photo or plaque in a central place
- Collecting money and making a donation to a favorite charity in the person's name
- Creating a scholarship fund
- Donating books to the library in memory of the deceased
- Planting a tree, bush or flowers
- Placing a piece of play equipment in the playground in honor of the deceased
- Writing a memorial piece for the yearbook
- Making a memorial book or video
- Crafting a memory quilt
- Setting up a grief center in the library
- Developing a memorial bird or wildlife garden area

Peer Support Groups

At The Dougy Center we have found that most children and teens respond well to peer support groups. Kids can help other kids, understand each other and share a common experience in ways adults can't. Dougy Center kids tell us that after a death they often can't talk to their friends or teachers about the death because they don't feel understood. Most kids tell us that grief groups are a very helpful resource, where they are able to share with others who have also experienced a death. In the support group the students do not feel different; they are like the other members. Students we talk to say it is helpful when the school provides support groups for students who have experienced the death of a special person.

You can also use peer support in the classroom to help students deal with and process their reactions to death. Because the grieving student does not want to be singled out or treated differently, it might be helpful to implement a class plan, including components of peer to peer, teams and cooperative learning.

One boy came to group and asked, "My mom wants to scatter some of my dad's ashes and keep some, is that weird?" He said his group was the only place he could ask such a question and not feel silly or crazy.

The peer model could team the grieving student with another student who has good listening skills and compassion, who can help the griever with assignments. This allows the griever to keep up with school work and stay successful in one area, when their world seems to be falling apart.

In a team-learning group, three or four students work together on a task. Each student has a part and contributes to the learning. The grieving student can be given a smaller part of the assignment. This gives the student a manageable piece to complete and a feeling of still being a successful part of the group.

A cooperative learning group includes the whole class as part of the learning process. Again, the amount of work assigned to the grieving student would be gauged by the amount of work that the student would be able to successfully complete under the circumstances.

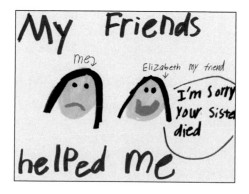

When a Teacher or Staff Person Dies

When a staff member dies, the whole school community is impacted. It is important to tell all the students about the death. Because individuals grieve differently, no one can predict how each student will respond. Having teachers watch out for high-risk students is helpful, but it is impossible to guess which student may have the most extreme reactions.

Students may exhibit varying reactions to the death of a school staff person, depending on how well they knew her, how the person died or other factors. Allowing the students to talk about the death and how they are being impacted by it is extremely helpful.

When a sixth-grade teacher died of a heart attack, the principal did not want to include the first and second graders in an assembly because he assumed that they did not really know her. We encouraged the school to include the younger children. Later they discovered that one 7 year old had been deeply affected because this teacher had walked by his house daily and they spoke to each other regularly.

When a Student Dies

When a student dies, the students in her classroom will be affected, but so will many others who are not in the class. Fellow team and club members, friends in other classes, boyfriends or girlfriends and classmates of siblings may all be grieving. No one can accurately predict who will and who won't be affected. We recommend that all students be given the same information, and that they all have the opportunity to see a counselor or go to a special "safe place" set up in the school for a period of time following a death.

When a Student's Family Member Dies

When a family member of one of your students dies, many of the same steps discussed in previous sections are useful. But in this case, the impact of the death may not touch as many students or teachers. The grieving student should be allowed to make choices about what is shared and how the information is shared with the class and school. Some students do not want to be treated differently and may not want the information shared at all. A student may want to tell the class herself or she may want the teacher to share the information. The student may want to be with the class or may choose not to be present when the teacher discusses the death. It is important to respect the wishes of the student.

10-year-old Amy kept a photo of her deceased father in her desk, and pulled it out when she needed extra support.

Students are usually very good about knowing what they need to do. It is most helpful for the teacher to talk to the student so that they can plan how to proceed together. They may decide that the student can put up a card when she needs to leave the area to be alone for a short time. The teacher may develop a "safe place" in the back of the room, the nurse's office or the library, where the student can spend some quiet time when needed.

Pet Death

Many students are affected by the death of a pet. Although pet deaths are not the same as the death of a person, they are an important part of the students' lives. Talking about and acknowledging the pet death provides the teacher with another "teachable moment" to discuss death and its impact on people. The teacher can discuss the difference between the death of a pet and the death of a person, and use this as an opportunity to discuss what death is. When a "classroom pet" dies, this too provides an opportunity for you and your students to talk about what happens when something or someone dies, and how they feel about it.

"Don't compare the death of your pet to a person's death, it's very different, not the same at all. You don't know how I feel after my brother's death if your cat died."

—Ben, 9

Special Considerations or Complications: Suicide, Homicide & Other Stigmatized Deaths

Many young children do not have a complete understanding of suicide, murder or other "stigmatized" deaths. They don't think of them as "better or worse" than a death by any other illness or accident. They simply focus on wishing the person were still alive. Others may understand and be able to process in a healthy way that the person died by suicide, AIDS or murder. Young children have not developed the "social condemnation" or stigma of suicide, AIDS deaths or homicide.

Unfortunately, our society tends to judge those who die by a death such as AIDS, suicide or murder. Often, their surviving family members are judged as well. Because of this, the grief of a stigmatized death tends to be complicated for the griever. In general, people do not know what to say or how to be around survivors of stigmatized deaths.

Because of their discomfort, they often stay away, not offering the same support they would if the death were from a car accident, cancer or other disease. This is very hard on the student and family, who often have little or no support after such a death.

It is important to tell the children and teens how the person died, using the appropriate words such as killed, murdered, shot, hung or

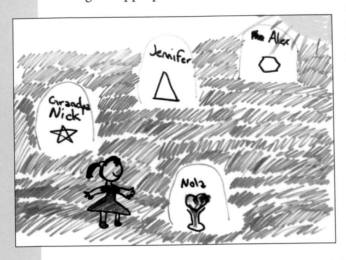

suicided. Although using these words with your students may be difficult, it is important for them to hear the truth from caring adults rather than from cruel students on the school grounds or on the evening news. After a sudden and violent death students may feel frightened and concerned about their own safety and the safety of those around them. Teachers may see increased absences of students, fear of getting to and from school and concern on the playground. There may be an increase in aggressive behavior and violent play. These students tend to become withdrawn from their peers.

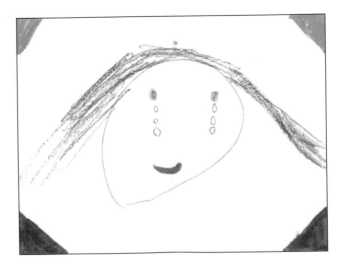

Death by Suicide

Death by suicide often evokes issues of abandonment, shame and social stigma. Students impacted by a suicide need to: understand that they are not alone; learn how to manage the anxiety that may result from the suicide; and have the opportunity to openly talk about why a person suicides.

In the case of a death by suicide, the surviving family members are often confused as to why the person died. They may experience guilt over not having prevented the death, or they may be extremely angry at the deceased for having taken his or her own life. Students affected by a suicide may have more chaotic energy or physical complaints, especially stomachaches. They often avoid the area where the death occurred and have fear of being alone. For some students there is a sense of relief at the death because of prior tension or anxiety that had surrounded the relationship with the deceased.

16 year old Toni reported that while standing at her locker between classes in the crowded hallway another student yelled at her, "No wonder your mother blew her brains out! I would too if I had a daughter like you!" A 10-year-old boy whose fighting on the playground consistently got him in trouble finally reported that the other kids were teasing him about his father's suicide.

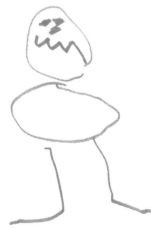

Because deaths by suicide are often judged harshly by our society, children and teens impacted by a suicide frequently do not want others to know how the person died. However, in most cases, people find out anyway. You should be alert for signs that the student is being teased or avoided by other students, and make an extra effort to provide support and understanding. Frequently children and teens who are acting out and have had a parent or sibling die by suicide are experiencing teasing from others.

If a student in your school dies by suicide, it is important to share that information honestly and forthrightly. Many adults are under the mistaken impression that talking about suicide will "put the idea in kid's minds," or increase the likelihood of an attempt.

Speaking honestly about this act, its consequences and impact on others may actually draw out students who are feeling suicidal and enable them to receive help. While many parents are uncomfortable with their children being exposed to the topic of suicide, it is important for children to hear the truth from trusted adults and educators. When a suicide occurs, students are talking about it among themselves, whether adults know it or not. It's better to share the factual information and provide help for hurting students rather than try to sweep it under the carpet.

Murder or Violent Death

Death from a murder often evokes issues of safety, loss of control, fear, rage, powerlessness and public humiliation. Children need to be able to share their fears and feelings of wanting revenge. They also need assistance in managing the anxiety that may result and to be given choices for accessing their own sense of control and power.

If children have witnessed a murder, they will have symptoms of trauma. Teachers will need information on these symptoms and will need to know how to respond. Those who are impacted by a death from homicide are often judged negatively by others. In an effort to protect themselves from believing that someone they love could be murdered, people sometimes believe that the family of the murder victim must have, in some way, contributed to the event. They feel safer if they think that "bad things only happen to bad people." Obviously this attitude alienates those who are impacted by a homicide.

Other factors that may make coping more difficult after a homicide are the impact of media attention, ongoing legal investigation and a potential trial. If the murderer is caught, there is someone to be angry with, but families seldom feel that justice has been done, no matter what the verdict is. Even if the accused is found guilty and sentenced to life in prison, that person gets to eat, breathe and sleep, while the person close to them who died doesn't.

If a suspect is never caught, many children and teens express fear that the person will come and harm them.

Death from AIDS

It has been our experience that students who have had a parent die of AIDS usually only share that their parent has died. They do not share how that person died, due to the social stigma associated with an AIDS death. Students may fear that if they do reveal that it was an AIDS-related death, they will be ostracized by the group. Because students in this situation tend to hold their feelings inside, they may experience a higher level of physical symptoms and concerns about their own health.

Death from Chronic Illness

When a family member's death is due to illness, students often develop issues around their own health. After such a death, children and teens want to share common experiences around the dying process. They want to talk about things like hospitalization, medical procedures, emergencies, changes in personality due to an illness and how illness affects relationships and social concerns. Students may also feel a sense of relief that the person died, because it means that they are no longer in pain.

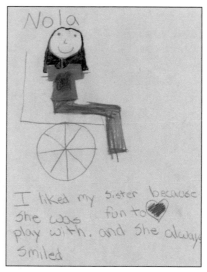

Accidental Death

Death from an accident often evokes issues of safety, loss of control, fear, powerlessness and unpredictability. Accidental deaths may occur in a variety of circumstances, including car accidents, work-related injuries, sports-related accidents, etc. Students need to share what they have been told about the accident and what they think actually happened. If the death was caused by a car crash, for example, and the student was involved, she will have symptoms of trauma. Teachers will need information on trauma symptoms and to know how to respond.

Deaths that Traumatize the School Community

When a death affects a large number of the staff and/or students, it becomes difficult for the school to adequately or appropriately deal with the impact. For example, if the principal is killed in an automobile accident, the entire school will be impacted. If, on a school outing, several children are injured and die in a school bus accident, the entire school community is affected. If an earthquake causes the gym wall to collapse and kills the basketball coach and several students, everyone is impacted. At these times it is important for the administration to recognize the impact and bring in outside help to process the death. The help could come from a neighboring school crisis team or the local mental health community.

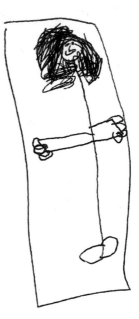

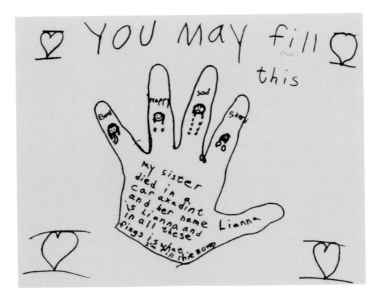

Classroom Activities to Help Students Deal with Grief

Activities can help your students express and deal with their grief. There are many things we have found helpful, including:

* Journal writing
* Art activities
* Reading books related to death
* Movement or dance activities
* Music
* Physical activities

The following activities are taken from the Memories Matter Activity Manuel. The manual consists of activities compiled by the staff and volunteers at The Dougy Center and are used in the groups conducted at the Center. Memories Matter is available through The Dougy Center's publishing division.

WHAT IS ALIVE? WHAT IS DEAD?

Age Level: 3 to 5 Years

Time Required: 45 Minutes to 1 Hour

Materials Needed: Various creatures and objects that are alive, dead and inanimate, book: Lifetimes, by Richard Tames

Goal: To help students distinguish between what is alive, dead and inanimate

Description of Activity:

1. Display various objects, one by one, in the center of the children's circle. Examples: a plant, toy animal, dead leaf, windup toy, live gerbil, doll, flashlight, warm water.

2. Have each child choose an item. Ask questions to give the children an opportunity to identify an object and tell why they chose it. Discuss what used to be alive, what is made of plastic, what the qualities of dead and alive are and what life is.
Examples: "Is something alive if it's warm?" (warm water) "Is something alive when it moves?" (windup toy)

3. Read the book Lifetimes and discuss the lifetimes of people and pets they have in their lives.

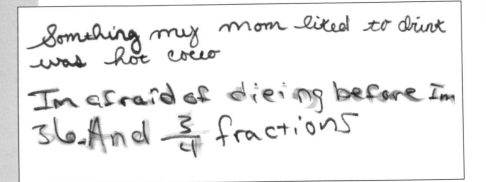

Something my mom liked to drink was hot coco

I'm afraid of dieing before I'm 36. And $\frac{3}{4}$ fractions

MEMORIALS, RITUALS AND FUNERALS

Age Level: 3 to 8 Years

Time Required: 30 Minutes

Materials Needed: Paper, crayons, felt pens, book: The Tenth Good Thing About Barney, by Judith Viorst.

Goal: To help students become more comfortable with funerals and memorials following the death of a loved one.

Description of Activity:

1. Read the book, The Tenth Good Thing About Barney.

2. Have the children list or draw things they remember about the person who died.

3. Discuss the funeral/memorial service of the deceased. Have the children discuss if they attended, what they remember, what were the best and worst parts for them.

4. Discuss the importance of remembering someone who died.

PARTING GIFTS

Age Level: 3 to 12 Years

Time Required: 15 to 30 Minutes

Materials Needed: Book: *Badger's Parting Gifts*, by Susan Varley, paper, crayons, liquid crayons and lapboards.

Goal: To remember the abilities taught to us by the person who died, to acknowledge that the person who died gave us lasting gifts and to remember them and have them with us always.

Description of Activity:

1. For younger students, tell the story of Badger's Parting Gifts or read the story as written.

2. Model an ability (i.e. whistling, skipping, climbing trees, singing, etc.) for the children that you learned from a person who died.

3. Invite the children to share abilities they were taught by the person who died. Examples:

Katie (5): "I can talk because my mommy talked to me. She helped me to learn to talk."

John (11): "My dad taught me how to shoot baskets. We went to the park almost every Saturday to shoot hoops. He was going to build a backboard for the driveway at our new house."

WHAT I REMEMBER MOST

Age Level: 4+ Years

Time Required: 10 Minutes

Materials Needed: Small plates, pens, paper, pencils, paints and brushes.

Goal: To give the students an opportunity to remember and share.

Description of Activity:

1. Have the students draw a circle on a piece of paper 8" x 10" or larger.

2. In the middle of the circle have them draw a picture of the person who died. Around the edges of the circle have them draw pictures and symbols or write words that remind them of that person.

3. Have students share their remembrances with the class.

MEMORY BOX

Age Level: 6+ Years

Time Required: 45 Minutes

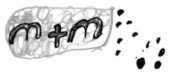

Materials Needed: Shoe boxes with lids, photos and personal items of the person who died, construction paper, magazines, fabric, scissors and glue.

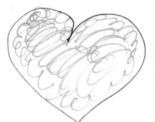

Goal: To help the students remember the deceased and have a safe place to put things that belonged to the deceased, as well as art or writings they make for that person.

Description of Activity:

1. Have the students decorate their box with materials, pictures and photos, etc.

2. Ask them to place memory objects, pictures, poems or written memories in the box.

3. Allow students to share with the group.

ANAGRAMS

Age Level: 7 to 18 Years

Time Required: 30 Minutes

Materials Needed: Paper and pens.

Goal: To remember and memorialize the person who died.

Description of Activity:

1. Have the children/teens write the name of the person who died vertically on a piece of paper.

2. The children/teens then write down words, sentences or phases which remind them of the person, using the letters of the name.

Examples:

TOM	LANA	FRANK
Tough	Loving	Funny
Outrageous	And	Round
Mighty	Never	Artistic
	Angry	Neat
		Knowing

3. Have the students share their remembrances.

BOOK OF THOUGHTS

Age Level: 6+ Years

Time Required: 30+ Minutes

Materials Needed: Paper folded in half to make a book, pencils, pens, markers and a stapler.

Goal: To facilitate journal-writing activities as a way of processing grief.

Description of Activity:

1. Each student is given a booklet of blank pages stapled together.

2. Ask the students to write one question or topic on the top of some of the pages that they would like to include in their Book of Thoughts.

Examples:
"One thing I would like to tell my mom." "One thing I would like to know about the person who died." Some of the pages can remain blank for writing whatever they are feeling.

3. The students can share their questions and topics with each other.

4. They then illustrate each topic page with a story, poem or drawing. Allow the students to have unfinished pages.

5. Have the students break up into small groups of two or three to share their books with others.

6. Encourage students to write daily in their journal.

MEMORY PICTURES

Age Level: All

Time Required: 30 to 45 Minutes

Materials Needed: Construction paper, magazines, index cards, colored pencils, crayons, metal rings, hole punch and snapshots (optional).

Goal: To acknowledge the experience of the students as real and valuable and to give them a way to share their feelings with classmates, family and friends.

Description of Activity:

1. Have the students connect 4" x 6" index cards or pieces of paper with a metal ring representing pages of a book.

2. They can then make a border for each page so the pictures will look like snapshots on the page.

3. The students will then draw memories and/or attach snapshots. They can use any media available to decorate the pages.

4. Encourage the students to share the book with family and friends whenever they feel ready.

Resources

Included here are a few of the books that the children, teens, parents and teachers find helpful. This is by no means an exhaustive list, but a few of their favorites or ones that help to teach and normalize the grief process for those who may not have the benefit of a support group.

Recommended Books for Children Ages 3 to 8

Brown, L.K. & M., *When Dinosaurs Die: Guide to Understanding Death*, Little Brown & Co., 1996 Douglas, E., *Rachel and the Upside Down Heart*, Price, Stern & Sloan, 1990

Mellonie, B. & Ingpen, R., *Lifetimes: A Beautiful Way to Explain Death to Children*, Bantam Books, 1983

Miles, R., *Annie and the Old One*, Little, Brown and Co., 1971

Old, W., *Stacy Had a Little Sister*, Albert Whitman & Co., 1995

Rogers, F., *When a Pet Dies*, GP Putman's Sons, 1988

Rothman, J., *A Birthday Present for Daniel: A Child's Story of Loss*, Prometheus Books, 1992

Sanford, D., *It Must Hurt A Lot: A Child's Book About Death*, Multnomah Press, 1986

Vorst, J., *The Tenth Good Thing About Barney*, Athenaeum, 1971

Virginia, J., *Saying Goodbye to Daddy*, Albert Whitman & Co., 1991

Recommended Books for Children Ages 9 to 12

Clifton, Lucille, *Everett Anderson's Goodbye*, Holt, Rinehart and Winston, 1988

Coburn, J. B., *Anne and the Sand Dobbies*, Harper Collins, 1980

Cohen, J., *I Had A Friend Named Peter: Talking to Children About the Death of a Friend*, William Morrow and Co., 1987

Cohen, J., *Why Did It Happen? Helping Children Cope in a Violent World*, Morrow Junior Books, 1994

Fine, J.C., *The Boy and the Dolphin*, Downeast Graphics, 1990

Krementz, Jill, *How It Feels When a Parent Dies*, Alfred A. Knopf, 1983

Levy, Erin, *Children Are Not Paper Dolls*, Harvest Printing, 1982

Madenski, M., *Some of the Pieces*, Little, Brown & Co., 1991

Mills, L., *The Rag Coat*, Little, Brown, & Co., 1991

Walker, A., *To Hell With Dying*, Hardcourt, Brace, Jovanovich, Pub., 1988

White, E. B., *Charlotte's Web*, Harper and Row, 195

Varley, S., *Badger's Parting Gifts*, Mulberry Books, 1984

Recommended Books for Children Ages 13 and Over

Fry, V., *A Part of Me Died Too*, Dutton Children's Books, 1995

Gootman, M.E., *When a Friend Dies: A Book for Teens about Grieving and Healing*, Free Spirit Publishing, 1994

Grollman, E., *Straight Talk About Death for Teenagers*, Beacon Press, 1993

Hipp, E., *Help for the Hard Times: Getting Through Loss*, Hazelden,1995

O'Toole, D., *Facing Change: Falling Apart and Coming Together in the Teen Years*, Mountain Rainbow Press, 1995

Paterson, K., *Bridge to Tarabithia*, Harper Collins, 1977

Recommended Reading for All Ages

Exupery, Antoine de Saint, *The Little Prince*, Harcourt, Brace, Javanovich

Hague, Michael, *The Velveteen Rabbit*, Holt, Rinehart, Winston

Lewis, C. S., *Chronicles of Narnia*, Macmillan (set of seven books)

Mandino, Og, and Kaye, Buddy, *The Gift of Acabar*, Bantam Books

Paulus, Trina, *Hope for the Flowers*, Paulist Press

Silverstein, Shel, *The Giving Tree*, Harper and Row

Additional Professional Resources

Adams, David W. and Deveau, Eleanor J. (ed), *Beyond the Innocence of Childhood*.

Baywood Publishing Co. Inc., *Helping Children and Adolescents Cope with Death and Bereavement*. Amityville, NY: 1995

Cassini, Kathleen K. and Rodgers, Jaqueline L., *Death and the Classroom: A Teachers Guide to Assist Grieving Students*. Cincinnati, OH: Griefworks of Cincinnati Inc., 1996

Fitzgerald, Helen, *The Grieving Child*. New York, NY: Fireside, 1992

Fox, Sandra Sutherland, *Good Grief: Helping Groups of Children When a Friend Dies*. Boston, MA: New England Association for the Education of Young Children, 1988

Gliko-Braden, Majel, *Grief Comes to the Classroom*. Omaha, NE: Centering Corporation, 1992

Goldman, Linda, *Breaking the Silence: A Guide to Help Children with Complicated Grief: Suicide, Homicide, AIDS, Violence and Abuse*. Bristol, PA: Taylor and Francis, 1996

Liotta, F.J., *When Students Grieve: A Guide to Bereavement in the Schools*. Horsham, PA: LPR Publisher, 1996

McEvoy, Alan W., *When Disaster Strikes: Preparing Schools for Bus Accidents, Murders, Suicides, Tornados and Other Community Catastrophies*. Holmes Beach, FL: Learning Publications Inc., 1992

O'Toole, D., *Growing Through Grief - A K-12 Curriculum*. Burnsville, NC: Compassion Books

Thomas, James T. ed., *Death and Dying in the Classroom*. Phoenix, AZ: Oryx Press, 1984

Ward, Barbara (ed)., *Good Grief: Exploring Feelings, Loss and Death with Over Elevens and Adults*. Bristol, PA: Jessica Kingsley Publisher, 1996

Webb, Nancy Boyd, *Helping Bereaved Children: A Handbook for Practitioners*. New York, NY: The Guilford Press, 1993

Wolfelt, Alan D., *Healing the Bereaved Child: Grief Gardening, Growth through Grief and other Touchstones for Caregivers*. Fort Collins, CO: Companion Press, 1996

Resources Also by the Dougy Center for Grieving Children

More in our Guidebook Series:

35 Ways to Help a Grieving Child

If you know a child or teen who has experienced a death, this guidebook presents you with simple and practical suggestions for how to support him or her. Learn what behaviors and reactions to expect from grieving children at different ages, ways to create safe outlets for children to express their thoughts and feelings, and how to be supportive during special events such as the memorial service, anniversaries and holidays. Available in English and Spanish.

Helping Children Cope with Death

This guidebook offers a comprehensive overview of how children grieve and strategies to support them. Based on The Dougy Center's work with thousands of grieving children and their families, you will learn how children understand death, how to talk with children about death at various developmental stages, how to be helpful, and when to seek outside help. This book is useful for parents, teachers, helping professionals and anyone trying to support a grieving child. Available in English and Spanish.

Helping Teens Cope with Death

This practical guide covers the unique grief responses of teenagers and the specific challenges they face. You will learn how death impacts teenagers, and ways that you can help them cope. The book also offers advice from parents and caregivers of bereaved teens on how to support adolescents and how to determine when professional help is needed. Available in English and Spanish.

What about the Kids? Understanding Their Needs in Funeral Planning & Services

This book addresses the best practices for funeral and memorial services with children and teens. Learn how to include children in these rituals and to involve them in the process. You will find suggestions from children and teens about what was helpful and unhelpful about the funeral or memorial service they attended.

When Death Impacts Your School: A Guide for School Administrators

A valuable resource for school personnel who are faced with a death or tragedy in their school community, this guidebook includes suggestions for how schools can help students—by addressing concerns, organizing memorials and offering support. It also includes instructions for developing a school intervention plan after a death, how to address issues related to suicide and violence, and how to decide when outside help is needed.

Activity Books:

After a Death: An Activity Book for Children

With a mixture of creative activities and tips for dealing with changes at school, home and with friends, this is a helpful tool for all grieving children. It includes a variety of drawing and writing exercises to help children remember the person who died, and learn new ways to live with the loss. Available in English and Spanish.

After a Suicide Death: An Activity Book for Grieving Kids

In this hands-on, interactive activity book, children who have had someone in their lives die of suicide can learn from other grieving kids. The workbook includes drawing activities, puzzles, stories, advice from other kids and helpful suggestions for navigating grief after a suicide death.

After a Murder: An Activity Book for Grieving Kids

Through the stories, thoughts and feelings of other kids who have had someone in their lives murdered, this hands-on workbook allows children to see that they are not alone in their feelings and experiences. The workbook includes drawing activities, puzzles and word games to help explain confusing elements specific to a murder, such as the police, media and legal system.

Memories Matter: 70 Activities for Grieving Children & Teens

Memories Matter features 70 activities to use with children and teens in peer support groups or for parents to use with their children. These activities are categorized by topic and are designed to help children process their unique grief.

DVDs:

Helping Teens Cope with Death

(21 minutes) is a window into the lives of six grieving teens who attended peer support groups at The Dougy Center. The DVD and 12-page companion guide provide insight to the thoughts, feelings, and changes that teens often experience. The DVD and guide are a resource for training purposes, or for general viewing by teens, parents, therapists, counselors and others.

Understanding Suicide, Supporting Children

(24 minutes) provides insight on the emotions and experiences that children, teens and families bereaved after a suicide death often go through, and offers ways to help. The DVD and 12-page companion guide are a resource for training purposes; for general viewing by children, teens, parents, therapists, counselors, professionals in the field of suicide prevention/postvention; and for anyone seeking to better understand suicide and how to support those grieving a suicide death.

Acting Out: The Scarlet D's on their Grief Trip
This documentary (75 minutes), produced by American Lifeograph Productions and filmed by Lani Jo Leigh, chronicles The Dougy Center's first Teen Theatre Troupe, The Scarlet D's, as they create, direct, and perform an original production about their experiences with grief. The DVD also includes complete footage of the Troupe's live performance (45 minutes). An emotionally engaging video, this is a powerful tool for grief support programs, schools, community groups, and families.

The above resources can be ordered by calling 503-775-5683 or through The Dougy Center's website at **www.dougy.org**.

What is The Dougy Center?

The mission of The Dougy Center is to provide loving support in a safe place where children, teens and their families who are grieving a death can share their experiences as they move through their healing processes. Through our National Center for Grieving Children & Families, we also provide support and training locally, nationally and internationally to individuals and organizations seeking to assist children and teens in grief.

The Dougy Center serves children and teens, ages 3 to 18, and young adults, 18 to 30 and their families who have experienced the death of a parent or sibling (or, in our teen groups, a friend), to accident, illness, suicide or murder. Peer grief support groups are provided and are coordinated by professional staff and trained volunteers. In addition, the parents or caregivers of the youth participate in support groups to address their needs and the issues of raising children following a traumatic loss.

When The Dougy Center was established in 1982, it was the first grief peer support program of its kind in the country. In response to numerous requests for information about our program, The Dougy Center has developed trainings and publications to help other communities establish centers for grieving children and families. Through our National Center for Grieving Children, The Dougy Center has trained individuals and groups throughout the world and publishes a National Directory of Children's Grief Services, updated annually.

The Dougy Center is a 501(c)3 nonprofit organization and raises its entire budget through contributions from individuals, businesses and foundations. We receive no federal funding or third-party payments. Participating families may contribute to the program, but there is no fee for service. While families receiving services contribute what they can, many do not have the financial resources to donate. Because The Center never turns a family away because of their inability to contribute, we are completely reliant upon private support from our friends in the community.

How can I support The Dougy Center or get additional information about its programs?

Contributions to The Dougy Center are tax-deductible to the full extent allowable under IRS guidelines. Your gift can be made to The Dougy Center on-line or mailed to us at the address below.

You can also receive additional information about:

- other guidebooks available from The Dougy Center
- videos and other resource materials available from The Dougy Center
- training for developing a children's grief center in your area
- the International Summer Institute held annually at The Dougy Center on developing a children's grief center in your area
- how to schedule a training or presentation in your area
- supporting The Dougy Center and its local and national programs to assist grieving children through a will or bequest

Write, call, fax or email:

The Dougy Center
P.O. Box 86852
Portland, OR 97286

503-775-5683
Fax: 503-777-3097

Email: help@dougy.org
Website: www.dougy.org

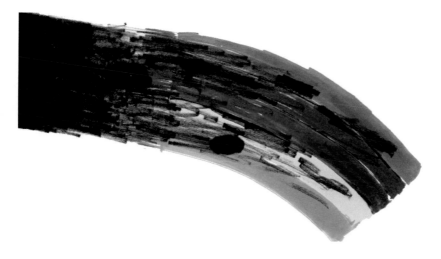

Contributors to this Guidebook include:

The Dougy Center staff:

Joan Schweizer Hoff, M.A.,

Program Director/Lead Writer

Donna L. Schuurman, Ed.D.,
National Director/Writing and Editing

Donald W. Spencer, M.Div., M.Ed., M.Coun.Psy.,
(former) Director of Family Services/Writing and Editing

Cover Art/Inside Art:
Provided by children from The Dougy Center

Design/Layout:
Fitzsimon GRAFIX/Fran Fitzsimon

The Dougy Center could not exist without the generous contributions of *hundreds of volunteers* who give of their time, boundless energy, unflagging enthusiasm and matchless dedication. We thank them for walking beside children and families on their journey of grieving.

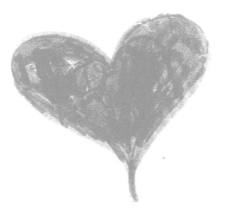

Notes

Made in the USA
Columbia, SC
20 June 2021